WELCOME

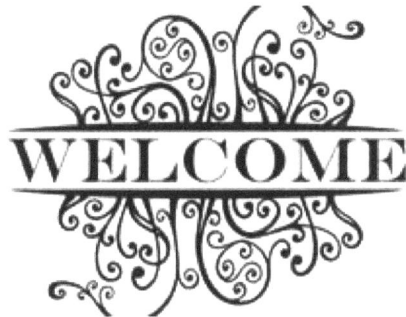

Welcome to a sample workshop of the I *Found My Voice Study Guide Series*. This sample is meant to give a snapshot of what the Participants can expect to learn when they attend the full workshop. The theme is finding one's own voice of authenticity, learning how to nurture it, self-discovery and steps for creating positive intentional change.

Have you ever wondered why you keep repeating the same defeating patterns in your life? Or how it is that you tend to attract unhealthy people into your life again and again? Perhaps you're stuck in the role your family gave you when you were coming up: the strong one, the good one, the pretty one, the smart one, the ugly one, the sick one, the weak one, the bad one, the not-so-smart-one, the always getting into trouble one—and you're ready to find your true identity now, without others telling you who you are.

Authenticity is the path to discovering the *real you*! Authenticity holds the mirror for you to look into, from the inside out. Authenticity is what you have been searching for, for a long time. Over the years, you seem to get little clues, make some progress, but it doesn't quite feel like, you've scratched the right spot yet.

I Found My Voice Study Guide 1: Workshop Sample
helps you experience self discovery as an informed adult.
It gives the Participant practical tools and steps to
complete fragmented stories of the past and to
confidently move forward in a balanced, healthy way.

Lastly the Guide allows you to tap into ongoing serenity
in a whole new way. Thanks for stopping by.

The Participants

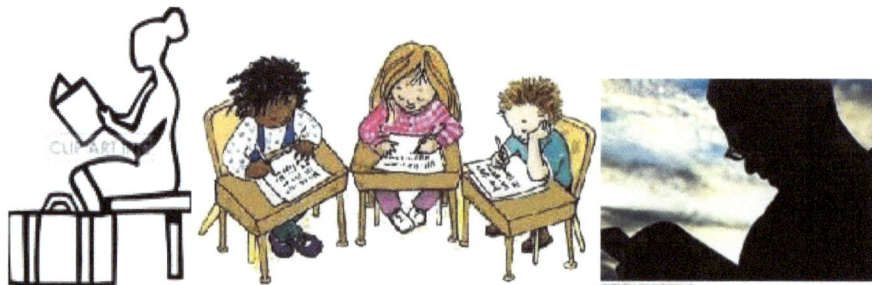

The Participants have the opportunity to tap into the Self and determine
what life goals are appropriate for the person they are now/becoming. The
workshop sets the stage, to begin to look at the questions: What still fits in
my life? What stays? What goes? How do I take better care of myself? Am I
Authentic? The Presentation should last for 30-60 minutes, depending on
the availability of the Participants, to get the full benefit of what the
workshop entails. This is an interactive workshop which promotes self-
discovery and basic steps for change. It is exciting, informative, and life
changing!

Welcome!

Dr. K

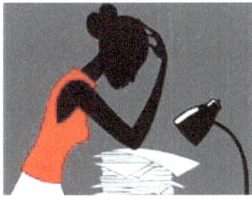

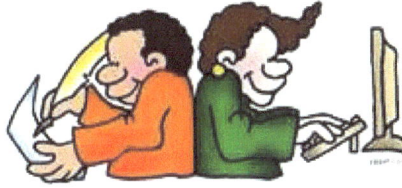

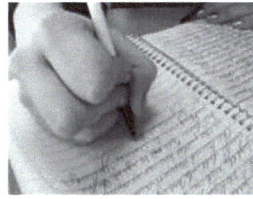

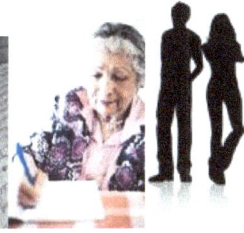

The Participant Objectives

The Participants will leave the Presentation with a practical and personal definition of Authenticity.

The Participants will initiate an Authenticity Statement.

The Participants will have the initial skill set to begin to examine their level of Authenticity in their daily lives and interactions.

The Participants will be able to state the value of Authenticity in their own words.

The Participants will be motivated to share this information with others.

The Purpose of the Guide

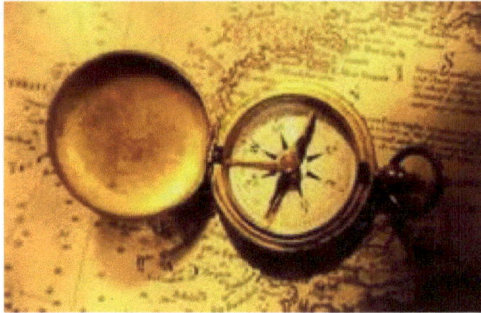

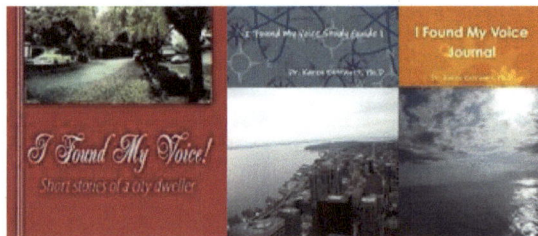

I Found My Voice Study Guide 1 is to be used in conjunction with *I Found My Voice!* and *I Found My Voice Journal.*(*www.Amazon.com or www. lulu.com.*)

In *I Found My Voice!* I describe my own journey of finding my voice. I reflect on the family and neighborhood I grew up in. Remembrances like Ms. Holly a retired woman who sponsored summer trips for all the neighborhood children. Social norms like everyone had the same dinner time, chores, homework and curfews. I describe through poetry and short stories, the people and experiences that greatly impacted my development, sense of security, and identity. Many of these "chance encounters" have influenced my choices, opinions, and actions as an adult. The theme for *I Found My Voice* ! is, reclaiming one's authenticity, valuing your own voice, nurturing the voice once it is claimed, and maintaining the Authentic You.

As I tell my stories about the unsung heroes/she-roes in my neighborhood, the reader has the opportunity to remember their own experiences of the people who shaped their lives. Within these memories are clues to the Original You.

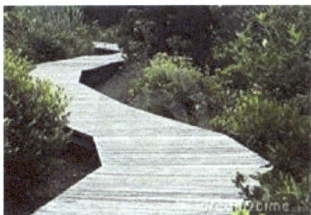

IFMVSG 1, gently guides you into your own path of discovery and re-discovery. We as adults have often become so busy with the "serious business of life" that we tend to forget sometimes, *how to Live!* Life is not meant to be a drudgery of paying bills, responsibilities, drone work, and collapsing into exhausted sleep cycles. Neither is it meant to solely scale the ladders of success by any means necessary, only to be lonely, disillusioned and surly when the pinnacle is reached.

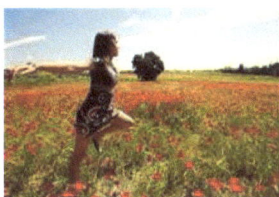

Chapter 1 begins with *Counting the Cost,* of self-discovery and change. Finding one's voice or Authenticity is a journey of experiences which seamlessly guide us to the people and circumstances which show us about the most important relationship we will ever have—the relationship with ourselves! How we interact with others is the mirror of how we love and care for ourselves, or not.

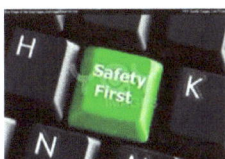

It is not usually an easy, soft paved road. The road is often filled with rough spots, gravel, and mud. It is the number one, transition process, which allows us to look at our integrity deficits with ourselves…It propels us to turn on the search light for ourselves.

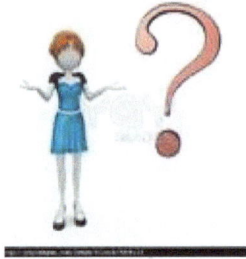

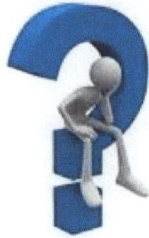

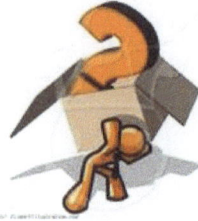

Authenticity is the ability to reframe the question of why do others treat me so bad to why do I allow myself to remain in situations which bring more sorrow than joy? What does this person teach me about how I treat and honor my own self-worth?

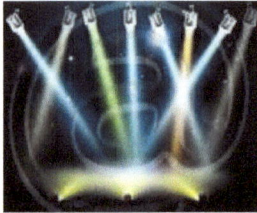

As the cliché says, *Life is truly a stage* and you get to choose which script you will enact for that day, season, or cycle. Life is all about the journey, learning new things about yourself first and others next.

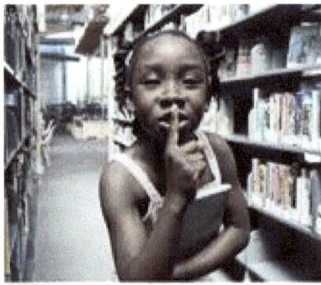

Pssst, sh-sh-sh—I want to let you in on some secrets, there is *not* just one destination in life! There is *not* that one thing that will happen and then your life will be PERFECT. There is *not* the one accomplishment that will cause you perpetual happiness. There is *not "the one" or "the thing'*—that will happen, occur, show up and then and only then will you be happy, successful, or have made it!

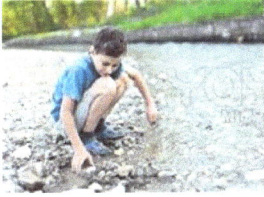

Instead there are ebbs and flows, every-day-occurrences, and plenty of opportunities to fall down, fall forward, get up, and stand still. Regardless of what it is, no one experience can represent all of life. *No matter what you've already encountered, whether you count it as good or bad or incidental. There is still so much more life to live!* To do this we must always be willing to practice going with the flow.

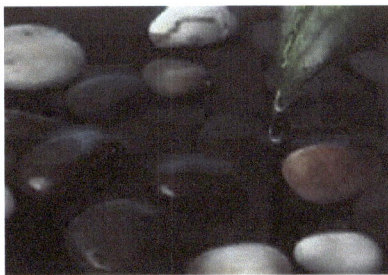

Attributes and Character can't show up if there's not anything to test or stretch you, not in some overly-stressful way, but in ways that continually give you the opportunity to choose growth or stagnation; life or death. The body/mind/spirit must have stimulation, new ground to step on, if you will.

Some of your best information about yourself will come through adversity, disappointment, mistakes, crises and unexpected circumstances; as well as poignant moments, belly-laughs with family and friends, music, dance, and all the shades of expression that you allow yourself to bring forth. This is the true nature of what Life is about. These are the times, when the real you will show up usually through your behaviors, opinions and how you respond.

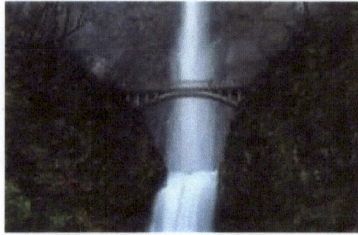

It is not fully possible to know whether you are a forgiving person unless you, have been betrayed, hurt, or lied to. The capability of being a seasoned, effective leader comes through allowing oneself to be a bridge for others to reach their potential. Bridges are suspended in air and rooted deep down in the bottom. Bridges allow movement, yet remain stable.

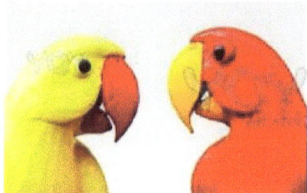

It is absolutely impossible to know and experience Love without being vulnerable, having misunderstandings, sharing who you are with someone else, and working through the changes of Life.

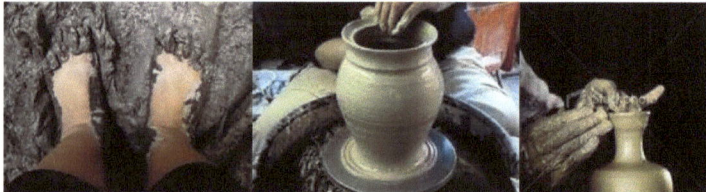

Sometimes we can get stuck and muddied by unresolved pain from the past or circumstances that did not turn out as one had expected. These are the times when New Clay must be gathered, water must be sprinkled and the hands guided in the making of a different vessel. This Study Guide is your personal invitation to come back to the things that create serenity and harmony within you; a beckoning to go find your potter's wheel and begin anew.

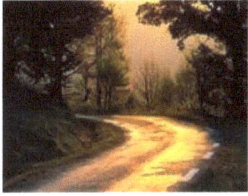

I Found My Voice Study Guide is an arrow pointing the way to the road that leads you to your own path. The Study Guide can get you on the road; however it is you who must decide whether you will allow your feet to step on your own path. Let us begin~

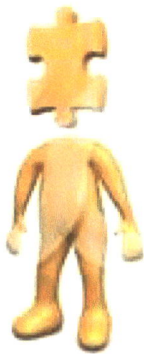

Authenticity: Will the Real Me, Please Stand Up!

Let's face it how many people do you meet on any given day that you can tell this is a person who is authentic, an individual, original and quite secure in their own personhood? I'm not talking about the arrogant, egotistical, gruff person that people scurry whenever they enter the room. I mean the person who you can just tell there's something about them—they seem to have a peaceful demeanor, a certainty, an extra dose of confidence that you rarely come across.

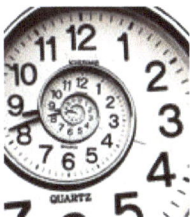

If there was a meter on you which registered how many times a day you make a decision or do something solely to please someone, or to be accepted or to appear that you belong to a particular status; what do you think it would show at the end of the day?

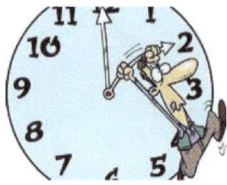

Likewise if there was a meter which registered how many times a day you were authentically you, what would the reading be at the end of the day?

There is always talk or advertisement about authentic jewelry, furniture, clothing, and so many other inanimate objects or expressions of materialism, but rarely do we take the time to consider Am I Authentic? Am I who I say I am? Or am I chameleon that changes all the time, depending on who's around?

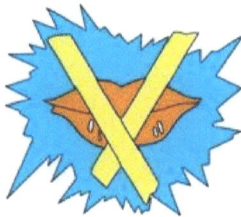

Do I speak my truth or do I pretend like it doesn't matter so I can stay in someone's good graces? Can I have an original thought or action or do I take my cues from others?

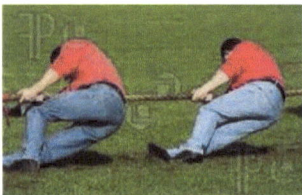

Over the years I have met many people who went into a career that the family, friends, and associates chose for them. They get the necessary education, training, or certifications required to do the work. They go in debt, miss out on social activities, and often make personal sacrifices in order to work in a field they did not choose! Often these are the people that hate their jobs, but feel like they *have to* stay because of what the response would be, if they walked away from this great opportunity that they never wanted!

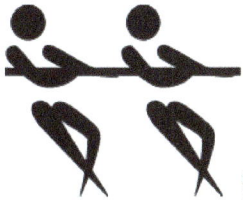

Same is true for people who date and marry the person their friends and family are impressed with, but not someone they love and feel they can make a life with. Yet, their need to please others or save face is stronger than their ability to be authentically who they are and make honorable choices for themselves.

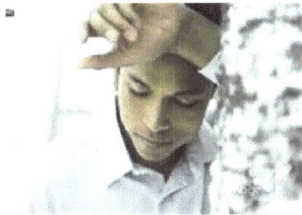

I remember a story a young co-worker told me many years ago. He talked about his college sweetheart, they never actually dated. They were more like friends. He said she had all the qualities that he was looking for in a wife and she was supportive of his dreams and he knew he could be very happy with this young lady. The only reason he did not pursue her or ask her to marry him was, she was full-figured and did not have sexy green eyes. Among his peers, a petite woman with green eyes and flowing hair was a status symbol—it meant he had arrived. He winced as he told this story about the one he wished he hadn't let get away. Although he was currently dating the petite woman with the sexy green eyes and flowing hair, he said he was miserable and wished he had had the courage to choose the woman that was right for him! He talked about how his friends were always patting him on the back and congratulating him for getting the status symbol of their group. *He described how happy they were for him and how miserable he was, living somebody else's dream!*

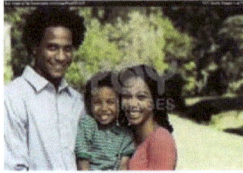

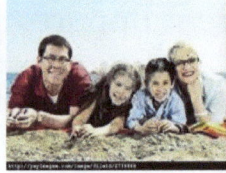

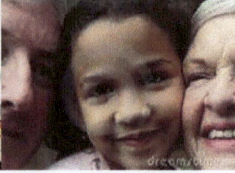

We all are shaped and form our identities through the people, places and things in our environment. This begins with the family or guardians who raise us and have great influence over our lives. After the family, social institutions like school, church, friends, economic status, gender, and ethnicity chime in to tell us who we are.

Child development says that almost all of our personality and identity is already formed by age 7. With so many different sets of hands on us, it is easy to see how our own personal authenticity could be marginalized, damaged, minimalized, and even erased. It's time to do an Authenticity Inventory.

For clarity sake, let's begin with the origin and definition of

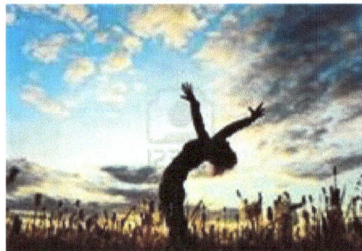

Authenticity:

What is Authenticity?

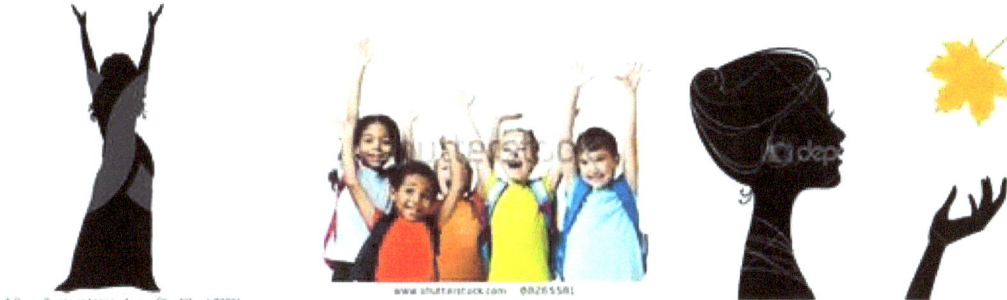

- *To be faithful to oneself, true to your own understanding of the world within first and then the world on the outside of you, next.*
- *To be sincerely dedicated and committed to the good intentions and attributes for oneself.*
- *To confidently stand in your own knowing of what is ideal, right, enriching, and honorable for you.*
- *To be able to produce original ideas, projects, and conclusions in a manner that brings forth life and creativity.*
- *To be free of the need to transform into a look, idea, career, marriage, friendship or anything else to please others at the cost of totally sacrificing yourself.*
- *To be unencumbered by society's standard of success when it does not match your own definition.*
- *To be clear of pretense or hypocrisy toward oneself or others.*

Children instinctively know how to be themselves. If they're hungry, have to go to the bathroom, tired, or happy you always know this is the real person. Most of us adults have forgotten how to be authentic and worse yet have forgotten the value of being who you are—to know it's OK to be who you are! Take note of the simplicity of a child, let the child teach you how to be genuinely-you!

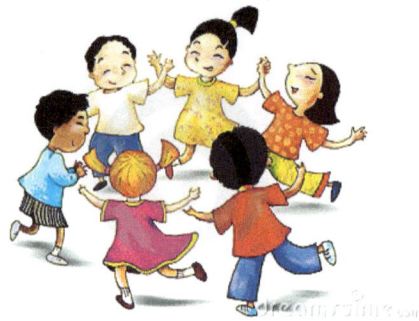

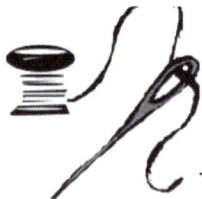

Yes adult life can have many challenging aspects to it and still, Authenticity must be the thread throughout one's life or we become the walking dead—devoid of emotions, compassion for self or others, cynical, and mean-spirited. You will have forgotten how to *enjoy life!*

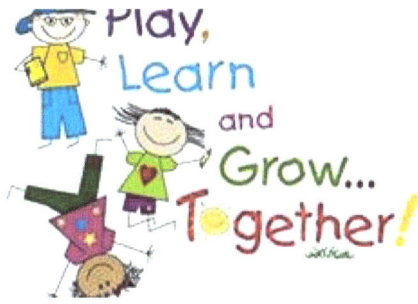

Exercise 0:

Just for a few minutes let's go back to a time when it is certain you were originally you. To complete this exercise you will need to remember yourself as a child, 7 years old or younger...

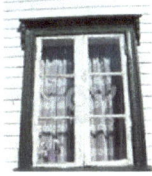What city and state did you live in? Who did you live with? What was your address, phone number, zip code?

_____
_____
_____
_____

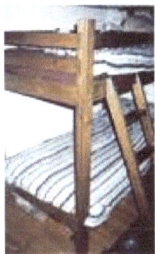

Describe your
bedroom_____
_____
_____
_____

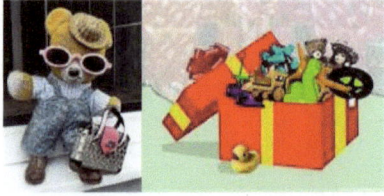

Name your favorite toy and how you got it.

_____

_____

_____

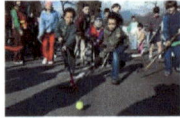

Name a friend and your favorite game.

_____

_____

Exercise 1:

You have 10 minutes to write a story including all of the above. Your story must have a minimum of 3 paragraphs. Begin!

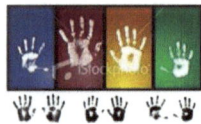

_____

_____

_____

_____

_____

_____

_____

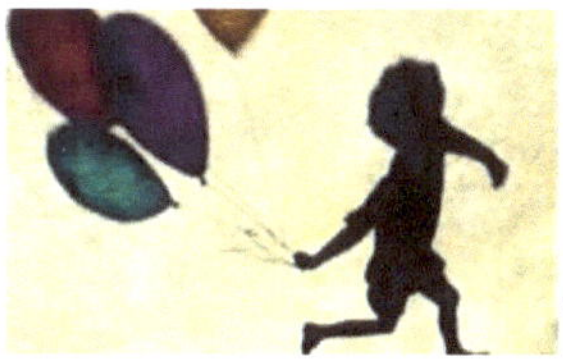

_____

_____

_____

_____

Exercise 2: You have 7 minutes to write how you feel about Authenticity and the memories Exercise 1 brought back.

_____

_____

_____

_____

_____

_____

_____

_____

_____

_____

_____

_____

_____

Authenticity Discussion

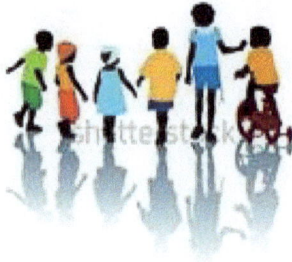

My Own Pledge

I Pledge allegiance to the

government of my own body & affairs.

Others opinions about it, I don't even care.

Why should I give this power to those outside of me?

Their opinions or stares are not a part of my destiny.

I look at them in amazement wondering, what makes them

Think they have authority over me?

I refuse to be defined by the category/boxes/labels of others.

Believe me, when I tell you I tried to fit in...to go w/ the

program...

To keep silent or pretend to nod, but the truth of the matter is, I was always the odd-man-out.

Whether they knew it or not, my real truth lied in my head & in my heart.

So now, it's OK if I don't make the A list or the B list.

It doesn't even matter if folks are un-comfortable with some Aspect of me.

The only thing that really counts is my own Pledge & Decree to be

Free in how I identify & look at me.

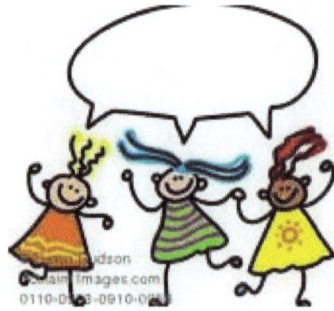

Feelings

After participating in the I Found My Voice Workshop sample

I feel_____

_____

_____

I've learned that My Authentic Self is

I_____

_____

_____

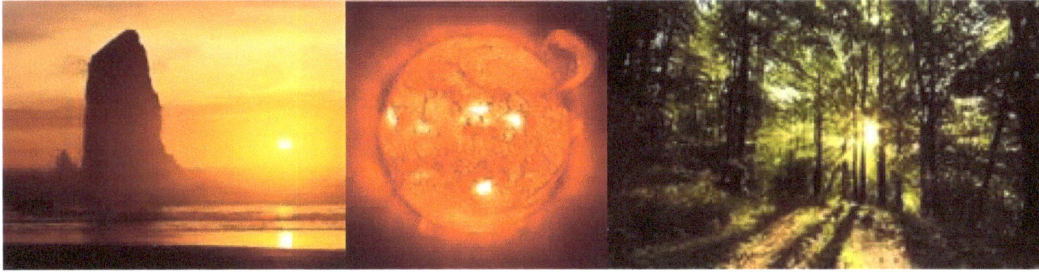

Here is my Decree for you:

May you be gently guided from darkness into the light of knowing better, doing better, and living better.

May your past pains and disappointments be stepping stones upon which character, integrity, and harmony come forth.

May you be able to let go what no longer works with grace and willingness of heart.

May laughter, good times, and close bonds surround you.

May you dwell in abundance of body, mind, spirit

and financial freedom;

All the days of your life and physical incarnation.

And so it is Indeed!

Dr. K

Originally You© Resources

Poems:

www.gspoetry.com (MHina)

Videos

Vimeo.com/Karen Entrantt

Baby Girle

Can Love Bring her Back

When a Woman Respects her Man

2 Artists 1 Love

A Love Conversation

Articles

http://www.allthingshealing.com/Poetry-Therapy/Poetry-is-MY-Therapy-Healing-Power-of-Your-Paper-Pen/8870#.Tkv_KeSSP-4.email

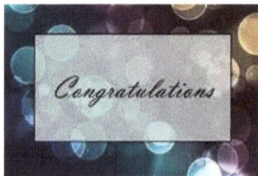

Congratulations

You have completed the Sample Workshop.

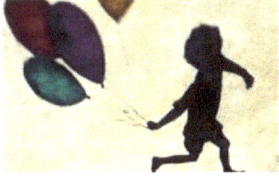

_____

_____

_____

_____

_____

_____

_____

_____

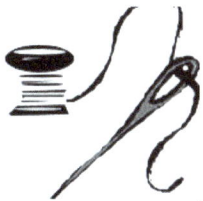 _____

_____

_____

_____

_____

_____

_____

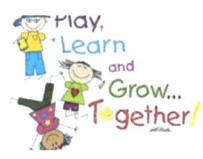

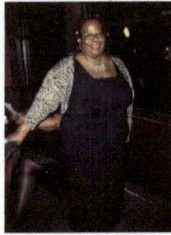

Dr. Karen Entrantt, Ph.D, who is lovingly referred to as Dr. K, is the Organizational Executive Director of GO GIRL Consults, A Life Coaching Company, which develops workshops and trainings. GO GIRL Consults is a licensed minority owned business. Dr. K has worked in the fields of Social Work, Mental Health, and Homelessness Prevention for over 33 years. As a well-seasoned Facilitator, she has the gift of reaching those who have almost given up on their dreams. She systematically demonstrates how every obstacle, disappointment or perceived set back can become a stepping stone to acquire the skills, patience, character, and determination to reach one's personal level of success.

Dr. K is passionate about helping others overcome obstacles and reach their personal goals. To attend one of her workshops is "an unforgettable, fantastic, life-changing experience!" As, many participants, state on their evaluation sheets. She uses her own real-world terms, strategies, humor, and interactive participation to help attendees become eager to embrace the next level of life expansion.

Dr. K is willing to bring these workshops to your meetings, gatherings, agency trainings, conferences, conventions, church and civic functions. Dr. K is also available to perform her life changing poetry at any event. Workshops can also be tailored to fit your specific group needs. K_poetry_seminars@yahoo.com

Dr. K is hard at work on several upcoming projects for release, which include: *I Found My Voice Study Guide 2*, which will be released in February 2013; : *I Found My Voice Study Guide 3*, which will be released in March 2013; *Finding the Depth of My Own Voice!* which is slated for release in April 2013. Her new *Children of Color Series* will be out in the Spring of 2013. This series will introduce several delightful children's characters who teach as they entertain and esteem children of color. *Weaning From Tradition to Nutrition*, is slated for release in the Fall of 2013.

Dr. K is also a story-teller and performing-poet. She has performed at The Act Theater, Seattle Town Hall, Westlake Mall and many other public and private venues.

www.ingramcontent.com/pod-product-compliance
Lightning Source LLC
Chambersburg PA
CBHW061059090426
42742CB00002B/96